GRAHAM E. TROPE

GLAUCOMA
A Patient's Guide
to the Disease,
Fourth Edition

UNIVERSITY OF TORONTO PRESS
Toronto Buffalo London

© University of Toronto Press 2011
Toronto Buffalo London
www.utppublishing.com
Printed in the U.S.A.

First edition printed 1997, 1999
Second edition printed 2001, 2003
Third edition printed 2004
Reprinted 2014

ISBN 978-0-8020-9473-5 (paper)

∞

Printed on acid-free paper

Library and Archives Canada Cataloguing in Publication

Trope, Graham E.
Glaucoma : a patient's guide to the disease /
Graham E. Trope. – 4th ed.

ISBN 978-0-8020-9473-5

1. Glaucoma – Popular works. 2. Glaucoma – Miscellanea. I. Title.

RE871.T76 2011   617.7′41   C2011-901247-2

Publication of this book has been made possible through a publication subsidy from Merck Canada Inc.

University of Toronto Press acknowledges the financial assistance to its publishing program of the Canada Council for the Arts and the Ontario Arts Council.

 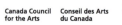

University of Toronto Press acknowledges the financial support of the Government of Canada through the Canada Book Fund for its publishing activities.

OPTH-1006467-0000

This book is dedicated to all patients who have taken the time to enquire about glaucoma, to the Glaucoma Research Society of Canada for the wonderful work they do to raise funds for glaucoma research, and especially to my wife, Angela, and children, Samantha and Matthew.

Contents

II TESTS FOR GLAUCOMA

III ALL ABOUT TREATMENT

Eye Drops

FIGURES

IV GLAUCOMA SOCIETIES

TRADEMARKS

Viagra™ is a trademark of Pfizer Canada Inc.

Avastin® is a trademark of Genentech, Inc.

Isopto® Carpine is a trademark of Alcon Canada Inc.

Phospholine Iodide® is a trademark of Storz; Division of Wyeth Ayerst Canada Inc.

Timoptic® and Timoptic-XE® Registered trademark of Merck Sharp & Dohme Corp., a subsidiary of Merck & Co., Inc. Used under license.

Betagan® is a trademark of Allergan Inc.

Betoptic® is a trademark of Alcon Canada Inc.

Iopidine® is a trademark of Alcon Canada Inc.

Alphagan™ and Alphagan P® are trademarks of Allergan Inc.

Trusopt® Registered trademark of Merck Sharp & Dohme Corp., a subsidiary of Merck & Co., Inc. Used under license.

Azopt® is a trademark of Alcon Canada Inc.

Xalatan™ and Xalacom® are trademarks of Pfizer Canada Inc.

Lumigan® and Lumgan® RC are trademarks of Allergan Inc.

Travatan® Z is a trademark of Alcon Canada Inc.

Taflotan® is a trademark of Santen Pharmaceutical Co., Ltd.

Cosopt® Registered trademark of Merck Sharp & Dohme Corp., a subsidiary of Merck & Co., Inc. Used under license.

Combigan® is a trademark of Allergan Inc.

Ganfort® is a trademark of Allergan Inc.

DuoTrav® is a trademark of Alcon Canada Inc.

Azarga® is a trademark of Alcon Canada Inc.

Diamox® and Neptazane® are trademarks of Storz; Division of Wyeth-Ayerst Canada Inc.

Preface

Glaucoma is unlike any other affliction. It usually causes no pain, discomfort, or distress. Central vision remains excellent until the very last stages of the condition. Patients are therefore often confused and initially reluctant to believe their vision is in danger. The purpose of this book is to inform patients about glaucoma, and to provide some insight into this condition. Information allows the patient to actively participate in the decision-making process along the long road to successful maintenance of vision.

This book was inspired by the thoughtful questions asked by numerous patients. Although there are excellent textbooks on glaucoma available in many libraries, they are written primarily for eye specialists, and can be difficult for the average person to obtain and understand. The Internet contains a lot of information on glaucoma but some of it is confusing and inaccurate. There is very little information available written in a straightforward manner for the patient suffering from glaucoma. The fourth edition of this book presents the latest information about the major aspects of glaucoma in a simple question-and-answer style.

My hope is that this book will provide you, the reader, with enough information to understand the disease so you can actively participate in the fight against humanity's major cause of irreversible blindness, glaucoma.

All about Glaucoma

1 / What is glaucoma?

Chronic open-angle glaucoma (also known as primary open-angle glaucoma) is a painless condition, often but not always associated with high pressure in the eye, which results in nerve damage and loss of vision. Normal pressure varies between 12 and 21 mmHg. Pressure is formed by fluid passing through the eye. This fluid, called the aqueous humour, is produced by a gland called the ciliary processes. The aqueous humour drains out of the eye through tissue in the front of the eye called the trabecular meshwork. The increased pressure causing glaucoma occurs when fluid flow through the eye's drainage system is obstructed (see figure 1, p. 77). High pressure is not always dangerous. In susceptible individuals, however, this high pressure does damage the eye, and in particular, the nerve at the back of the eye (see figure 2, p. 78). The nerve becomes 'cupped' and eventually the vision starts to fail. The loss of peripheral or side vision is characteristic of glaucoma. Central vision is typically not affected until very late in the disease process.

2 / What are the basic parts of the eye?

Knowing a few basic facts about the eye and how it works will give you a better understanding of glaucoma and how it affects you.

The outer layer of the eyeball is called the sclera. This thin yet tough protective shell is the white of the eye and is covered by a transparent membrane called the conjunctiva. The front part of the sclera is known as the cornea. This is the clear tissue through which light enters the eye. The coloured portion of the eye is the iris. It contains muscles that control the size of the pupil, which is the dark-coloured area in the centre of the iris. The muscles of the iris regulate how much light enters the eye, and depending on the amount of light, the pupil responds by becoming bigger (dilating) or smaller (constricting). The lens of the eye is located behind the iris. It changes its shape to focus images onto the retina – the area at the back of the eye. The retina delivers the images to the brain via nerve signals sent through the optic nerve. All these different parts work together to produce signals which are sent to the brain to produce a visual image or picture.

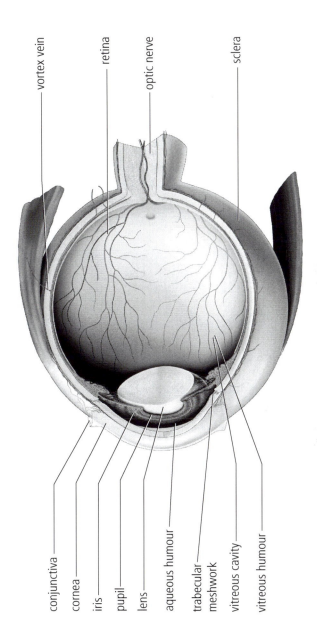

vortex vein

retina

optic nerve

sclera

conjunctiva

cornea

iris

pupil

lens

aqueous humour

trabecular meshwork

vitreous cavity

vitreous humour

The inside of the eye is filled with fluid. The centre of the eye, called the vitreous cavity, is filled with a gel-like substance called vitreous humour. The front compartment of the eye (bounded by the cornea, iris, pupil, and lens) is filled with a watery fluid called the aqueous humour. This special fluid is responsible for the pressure we measure in the eye. This pressure is known as the intraocular pressure (IOP).

3 / What are the names of the different types of glaucoma?

There are a variety of glaucoma types. These include:

1) Primary or chronic open-angle glaucoma (including low or normal pressure glaucoma)
2) Primary angle-closure glaucoma
3) Secondary open-angle glaucoma, including:
    - Steroid-induced glaucoma
    - Pseudoexfoliation
    - Pigmentary glaucoma
    - Uveitic glaucoma
    - Angle recession (trauma)
4) Secondary closed-angle glaucoma, including:
    - Neovascular glaucoma
    - ICE Syndrome

5) Congenital glaucoma.

Of all the different types of glaucoma, the most common is primary or chronic open-angle glaucoma. It accounts for approximately 90 per cent of all cases in Caucasians. Primary angle-closure glaucoma is the painful form of the disease that is also often called acute glaucoma. Primary angle-closure glaucoma is much more common in Asian than in Caucasian eyes.

4 / What is the difference between glaucoma and ocular hypertension?

Glaucoma refers specifically to damage to the optic nerve and/or the peripheral vision. Ocular hypertension refers to high pressure which does not damage the nerve or vision. Patients with ocular hypertension are often called glaucoma suspects. Most glaucoma suspects do not go on to develop glaucomatous nerve and vision damage.

5 / My doctor says I am a glaucoma suspect. What does this mean?

The term glaucoma suspect often refers to a patient with high eye pressure but without damage to the optic nerve or visual field. Most patients with ocular hypertension do not require treatment, and will not get glaucoma. However, about 33 per cent of patients with high pressure do eventually go on to develop glaucomatous damage. As a result it is absolutely essential that glaucoma suspects be examined at least once a year to rule out the development of early damage and the need for therapy.

6 / What is normal eye pressure?

Normal eye pressure is between 12 and 21 millimetres of mercury (mmHg), with average pressure being 15.5 mmHg. Pressure above 21 mmHg is considered abnormal. Damage, however, can occur at different pressures in different individuals. Some patients develop glaucomatous nerve damage at pressures far below 21 mmHg, while others develop nerve damage only at very high pressures. Your eye specialist will tell you whether your pressure is normal for you as an individual.

7 / With glaucoma, what happens to the intraocular pressure in the eye?

In a healthy person, the eye's fluid or aqueous humour continuously drains through an area called the trabecular meshwork to maintain normal pressure. In many patients with glaucoma, the pressure in the eye builds up and rises because there is damage to the drainage system. For example, in chronic open-angle glaucoma, the trabecular meshwork blocks outflow of fluid (see green arrow in figure 1), so that fluid accumulates, increasing pressure that can gradually damage the optic nerve.

8 / Can I develop glaucoma without having an increase in eye pressure?

Research shows that in about a third of patients with glaucoma, there is little or no increase in eye pressure or ocular hypertension (this is called normal pressure or low tension glaucoma). But the exact cause for glaucoma in these patients is still unknown. Although pressure still plays a role in causing this form of glaucoma, there are likely other factors involved, such as blood flow, low blood pressure, or optic nerve biomechanical weakness. Lowering eye pressure has been shown to prevent deterioration in patients with normal tension glaucoma.

9 / How common is glaucoma?

Approximately 67 million people worldwide have glaucoma. In Canada, more than 300,000 people are affected. The most common type seen in North Americans is chronic or primary open-angle glaucoma. In Asia angle-closure glaucoma is the most common type of glaucoma. Glaucoma is the second most common cause of blindness. For every person blinded by glaucoma, six others have lost useful vision in one eye. To prevent serious problems, see your eye doctor for regular eye exams every year.

10 / I see very well and do not wear glasses. How can I have glaucoma?

It is important to remember that glaucoma does not affect your central vision. Glaucoma affects side vision first, and only affects central vision very late in the disease. Therefore, glaucoma has no effect at all on your need to wear glasses.

11/ Does glaucoma cause blindness?

Glaucoma is the most common cause of preventable blindness. That is why regular eye examinations are so important. If glaucoma is treated promptly, it can usually be controlled and vision saved.

12 / Can my children inherit glaucoma from me?

Yes, this is possible, although not always the case. Children whose parents have glaucoma have a much greater risk for the disease and should have annual eye examinations after the age of 18. A defect has been discovered in the TIGR (myocilin) gene. It is found in an unusual form of juvenile (under 30 years) glaucoma. Other defects have also been found in babies born with glaucoma (see question 45). However, genetic defects have not as yet been found in the most common type of glaucoma called chronic open-angle glaucoma.

13 / Is glaucoma contagious?

No, it is not an infectious disease.

14 / Is glaucoma caused by stress?

No. Unlike blood pressure, eye pressure is relatively unaffected by stress.

15 / What is cupping of the optic nerve?

The optic nerve at the back of your eye carries all of the visual stimuli to the brain. The normal optic nerve looks a bit like a doughnut. It has a pale central area called the cup. The rim surrounds the cup and is the part of the nerve carrying the electrical impulses from the eye to the brain. In glaucoma the rim gets thinner and the pale cup area gets bigger. This process is known as cupping. If your doctor says your nerve is cupped, this means your nerve is damaged, with an enlarged central cup and thin rim (see figure 2).

16 / How do I know if my optic nerve is damaged from glaucoma?

The normal optic nerve has a small pale central area known as the cup (see question 15 and figure 2). In glaucoma this cup (or cupping) enlarges to more than 70 per cent of the entire nerve. The ratio of the cup to the entire nerve is known as the cup to disk ratio. It is important for you to ask your eye doctor to tell you about your cup to disk ratio. If it is more than 70 per cent (or 0.7) then your nerve is likely damaged from glaucoma. In very severe glaucoma this cupping can damage the whole nerve. In glaucoma that is getting worse, progressive cupping (your cup to disk ratio gets larger, for example, going from 0.7 to 0.85) means your glaucoma is deteriorating. Sometimes in glaucoma just small parts of the nerve are damaged. This is known as notching. Notching is commonly seen in low pressure glaucoma (see question 8). Other signs of nerve damage include a hemorrhage on the nerve (see question 17 and figure 2). It is important to know that in most patients nerve damage develops before visual field damage. The informed patient will therefore want to know if the nerve is damaged (ask for your cup to disk ratio) and the results of the visual field test (see question 6 under Tests for Glaucoma).

17 / My doctor says there is a hemorrhage on my nerve. What does this mean?

In glaucoma a small hemorrhage can, on occasion, be seen on the rim of the optic nerve (see figure 2). This hemorrhage indicates that the pressure is too high for the optic nerve. If a hemorrhage is found, your eye specialist will usually recommend lowering your pressure to a safer level with eye drops, laser treatment, or surgery.

18 / What are the risk factors for glaucoma?

Individuals who are more likely to be at risk are:

1) Over age fifty
2) Related to someone with glaucoma
3) Of African descent
4) Very short-sighted
5) Have high eye pressure and large fluctuations in daily eye pressure
6) Have a thin cornea
7) Have a disc hemorrhage
8) Have disc asymmetry

Perhaps the most important of these are high eye pressure and being related to someone with glaucoma. Glaucoma is unusual in people under the age of fifty. It is more common in patients with a strong family history and in those who are very short-sighted. African Americans are three times as likely to develop glaucoma as are whites of the same age. There is also a slight increase in glaucoma in patients who suffer from diabetes.

19 / Does glaucoma cause high blood pressure?

No. Having glaucoma will not increase your blood pressure.

20 / If my blood pressure is high, will my eye pressure be high?

Not necessarily. Although there is an indirect relationship between high blood pressure and glaucoma in older patients, patients under stress or who experience a sudden increase in blood pressure do not usually have high eye pressure.

21 / Does glaucoma produce eye strain and headaches?

No. Chronic glaucoma is symptomless. Most patients do not know they have the disease.

22 / Should I avoid over-the-counter medications if I have chronic glaucoma?

Over-the-counter medications should be avoided only if your eye specialist tells you that your angle is narrow; that is, that you are at risk of angle-closure glaucoma – an unusual form of glaucoma in Caucasians. Prescription drugs may indicate on the package insert that they should not be used by patients with glaucoma. What is really meant is that patients at risk of angle-closure glaucoma should not use the medication as the drug may dilate the pupil, resulting in acute glaucoma. Ask your eye doctor to explain the type of glaucoma you have. Generally, patients with chronic open-angle glaucoma can use prescription and non-prescription drugs as none of these have adverse effects in relation to glaucoma. The exception to this rule is steroids (cortisone), which, in oral, eye-drop, inhaled, topical, and injected forms, can aggravate chronic glaucoma.

23 / Some patients with glaucoma feel pain. Is this common?

Glaucoma patients who feel pain suffer from acute glaucoma, an unusual form of glaucoma. Patients may have loss of vision, severe pain, a red eye, nausea and vomiting, and very high intraocular pressure. Sometimes before the attack begins patients will see haloes around lights. This condition requires immediate eye-drop treatment, followed by laser treatment (see figure 3, p. 79).

24 / What is the cause of acute glaucoma?

Acute glaucoma is caused by the sudden closure of the drainage channels by the iris (the colored part of the eye). This type of glaucoma is cured by laser treatment to the iris. Cataract surgery may be advised in some cases as lenses that have enlarged with age seem to play a role in causing the problem (see figure 3).

25 / Does open-angle glaucoma cause cataracts?

There is no relationship between glaucoma

and cataracts. However, as glaucoma and cataracts both tend to occur in older patients, they often appear around the same time.

26 / Does caffeine make glaucoma worse?

Although some studies have indicated that caffeine has an effect on glaucoma, most of the recent studies suggest that drinking coffee and/or tea in moderation will not unduly influence your glaucoma.

27 / Will I go blind from glaucoma?

If diagnosed and treated early, glaucoma will not usually produce blindness. Although glaucoma does slowly progress in many patients, glaucoma usually does not cause blindness if treated aggressively.

28 / Can vision deteriorate despite treatment for glaucoma?

Yes. As we get older, we lose cells in the optic nerve responsible for vision. This is part of the normal aging process. Patients with severe damage from glaucoma will be more aware of this progressive loss of vision. At the present time there is nothing that can be done about this change due to aging. It is therefore essential that glaucoma be diagnosed early before damage occurs to the nerve cells.

29 / Who diagnoses and treats glaucoma?

Glaucoma is usually discovered during a routine eye examination performed by an optometrist or ophthalmologist. All ophthalmologists and some optometrists are licensed to treat glaucoma with eye drops. Laser treatment and surgery are usually carried out by an ophthalmologist. Your eye specialist may refer you to a glaucoma specialist if there is doubt about the diagnosis or if there is need for further care.

30 / Will my glaucoma ever go away?

No. Glaucoma never goes away. Even the very best treatment does not reverse damage from this disease. The best we can do currently is to control glaucoma with eye drops, laser treatment, or surgery.

31 / Is any research being done to promote early diagnosis of glaucoma?

Yes. Much research is currently being done on the development of tests to enable us to diagnose damage at an earlier stage. These tests include newer imaging techniques, new vision tests, and electrophysiological tests.

32 / Are there any popular misconceptions about glaucoma?

The majority of North Americans have the mistaken belief that vision lost to glaucoma can be restored. In one survey approximately 54 per cent of North Americans indicated that they believe that eye damage from glaucoma can be corrected. As well, 53 per cent reported that they believe that in the early stages of glaucoma, one can feel increased pressure in the eyes. Although these beliefs are common, they are mistaken.

33 / In the early stages of glaucoma can I feel pressure in my eye?

No. Chronic glaucoma causes vision loss without warning symptoms. (See question 32.)

34 / Does glaucoma commonly cause blindness in African Americans?

Yes. Glaucoma is the most common cause of blindness in individuals of African origin. African–North Americans are at least three times as likely to develop glaucoma damage as are whites of the same age.

35 / Does emotional stress affect my intraocular pressure?

There is no scientific evidence to suggest that emotional stress affects intraocular pressure.

36 / Can lack of sleep or emotional stress associated with the visual field test push my pressure up on the day of the eye examination?

There is no evidence to suggest that lack of

sleep the night before an examination or anxiety about the eye exam or the visual field test can change eye pressure.

37 / Will changing my diet or taking herbs help my glaucoma?

No. There is no evidence that changing one's diet will influence glaucoma. There is also no evidence that taking herbs (such as bilberry) influences glaucoma. Vitamin C and minerals including magnesium and chromium have not been shown to help glaucoma. Ginkgo biloba has been shown to improve blood flow to the brain. Its influence on glaucoma, however, is not known.

38 / Does smoking or drinking alcohol have an impact on my glaucoma?

Neither alcohol use nor smoking causes glaucoma, although alcohol can lower intraocular pressure for a few hours under certain conditions.

39 / My eyes feel gritty and tender. Is this a result of the high pressure from glaucoma?

No. Chronic glaucoma has absolutely no symptoms at all. Grittiness is often caused by dry eyes, a condition which can be made worse by use of glaucoma eye drops. Artificial teardrops, particularly those without preservative, can often relieve gritty eyes caused by lack of tears.

40 / Will sexual activity affect my glaucoma?

No. Sexual activity has no positive or negative effect on glaucoma.

41 / Does Viagra™ (Sildenafil Citrate) improve or worsen glaucoma?

Viagra and other similar erection-promoting drugs have not been shown to worsen or improve glaucoma. They have been reported to produce coloured or 'blue' vision. To date there are no reports that the medications adversely affect blood flow to the eye in patients with glaucoma.

42 / What is congenital glaucoma?

Primary congenital glaucoma results from the abnormal development of the structures forming the front of the eye. It develops before the age of three and is usually diagnosed at birth or shortly thereafter. Most cases are recognized during the first year of life. This type of glaucoma affects both eyes. It is very rare but can run in families. Genetic testing has identified abnormal genes in some families with this disease. See question 45 for further information.

43 / What is developmental glaucoma?

Some children and young adults can develop glaucoma associated with other bodily abnormalities. These conditions have strange-sounding names such as Axenfeldt-Reigers syndrome and Aniridia. Developmental glaucomas like Axenfeldt often run in families and can be associated with other conditions such as small or short teeth, facial flattening, or a protruding lower lip. In the condition Aniridia the child often has no iris and therefore no eye color. These children often have poor vision. Children with developmental glaucomas usually develop glaucoma after the age of three, often during the teenage years. All developmental glaucomas have high pressure due to blockage of the drainage system from abnormal eye development. Pressure in the eye must be lowered with drops or surgery in all forms of developmental glaucoma to protect the optic nerve from damage.

44 / What is juvenile glaucoma?

Juvenile glaucoma is an inherited form of glaucoma that develops at a much earlier age than primary open-angle/chronic glaucoma. Juvenile glaucoma can occur in older children, young teenagers, or young adults. A number of genetic abnormalities have been described in some people with juvenile glaucoma. This disease is very similar to the adult form of open-angle glaucoma but the intraocular pressure is often very high. As with the adult form of glaucoma the problem is due to a blockage in the drainage system. Treatment includes eye drops and, if necessary, surgery. Laser treatment does not usually work in patients with juvenile glaucoma.

45 / Can babies be born with glaucoma?

Yes, babies can be born with or develop congenital glaucoma (see question 42). This very rare form of glaucoma is characterized by tearing, enlargement of the front of the eye, and sensitivity to light. This condition is not related to the more common chronic open-angle glaucoma experienced by adults. Similarities, however, include an increase in pressure in the eye. In a baby this is due to poor development of the drainage system. Unlike the treatment of adult forms of glaucoma, treatment of congenital glaucoma is always surgery.

46 / How does chronic glaucoma differ from other glaucomas?

In Caucasians and African Americans chronic open-angle glaucoma is by far the most common form of glaucoma. It occurs in older patients and is due to poor drainage of fluid from the eye. There are, however, many other causes of glaucoma – all due to blockage of the drainage system in the angle of the eye. These rare forms of glaucoma can be caused by new vessels (seen in patients with diabetes or with blockage of a blood vessel in the eye), inflammatory material (seen in patients with a condition called uveitis or iritis), pigment granules from the iris (seen in patients with pigmentary glaucoma), or a dandruff-like material in a condition known as pseudoexfoliation. Trauma to the eyeball can also cause glaucoma by damaging the drainage system.

47 / Is eye pressure affected by menopause?

There is no evidence that menopause either raises or lowers eye pressure, or that menopause affects glaucoma.

48 / My distance vision has deteriorated a lot in the past few months. Is this due to glaucoma?

Glaucoma does not affect distance vision. Pilocarpine (an eye drop sometimes used to treat glaucoma) can make the pupil so small that inadequate amounts of light get into the eye. This can lead to decreased vision, particularly in a dark room.

49 / My eyeball hurts when I read. Does eye strain cause glaucoma?

No. Eye strain and reading do not cause or worsen glaucoma.

50 / Can a blow to the eye cause glaucoma?

Trauma to the eye can lead to the development of glaucoma, when damage has been done to the drainage system (the trabecular meshwork). If you have received a hard blow to the eye, you should be examined regularly to rule out the possible development of glaucoma or retinal detachment.

51 / What is pseudoexfoliation?

Pseudoexfoliation is the shedding of a flaky white material found throughout the eye. It is best seen on the lens. Its presence is often associated with an aggressive form of glaucoma. Patients with pseudoexfoliative glaucoma often have very high eye pressure, which can be more difficult to control. This type of glaucoma responds to the usual therapies, including laser trabeculoplasty.

52 / What is pigmentary glaucoma?

Pigmentary glaucoma is an unusual form of glaucoma occurring in young, often short-sighted adults. It is characterized by the presence of pigment granules throughout the eye, which block the drainage system. Occasionally the pigment can cause blurred vision during vigorous exercise. As is the case in patients suffering from pseudoexfoliation (see question 51), pressure is often high in the eyes of those with pigmentary glaucoma. This type of glaucoma responds well to the usual treatment, including laser treatment.

53 / What is neovascular glaucoma?

Neovascular glaucoma forms when new vessels in the angle of the eye block the drainage system. These vessels are associated with a number of conditions, including diabetes, after blockage of a blood vessel at the back of the eye (retinal vein occlusion), or when there is poor blood supply to the eye. In diabetics this type of glaucoma can be prevented by good blood sugar control, use of newer drugs like Avastin® (Bevacizumab), and laser treatment. This glaucoma is difficult to treat when the drainage angle has closed off leading to high eye pressure. We attempt to treat this condition with eye drops, laser treatment, and often eye surgery. Vision is often poor in patients with this condition.

54 / What is steroid-induced glaucoma?

This is a form of glaucoma initiated or worsened by use of steroid inhalers, tablets, and injections, but especially by steroid eye drops. Glaucoma patients and their families are at greater risk of a pressure increase from steroid use. Patients with glaucoma should never use steroids in any form unless under the direction of an eye specialist.

55 / Can I do anything to help my glaucoma?

Regular exercise can lower eye pressure and help glaucoma. Never use steroid (cortisone) eye drops, tablets, or lung inhalers without your glaucoma doctor's supervision. All steroids (except for the occasional injection into an arthritic joint) make glaucoma worse. It usually takes about two weeks of steroid use to increase eye pressure.

Don't drink huge amounts of water or beverages like beer (over 8 large glasses per day). Too much fluid can overload your drainage system and increase eye pressure. If you do yoga never stand on your head because this increases eye pressure. Glaucoma sufferers should also avoid playing wind instruments like the trumpet as blowing very hard for long periods of time can increase eye pressure.

Some reports indicate tight shirt collars and ties can increase the eye pressure. Do not wear a tight tie if you suffer from chronic glaucoma and never wear neck compressing deep sea diving equipment if you have glaucoma.

Tests for Glaucoma

1 / How often should I undergo testing for glaucoma?

If your glaucoma is well controlled, most ophthalmologists recommend twice-yearly eye exams.

2 / Are any of the tests for glaucoma painful?

No. The tests include a pressure test of the eyes, a field of vision test (which tests peripheral vision), imaging tests, and an eye examination.

3 / Why does my ophthalmologist use drops to enlarge my pupils? Can this damage my eyes?

Your ophthalmologist will dilate your pupils so that he or she can get a good look at the optic nerve at the back of the eyes. Careful examination of the optic nerve head will indicate to the ophthalmologist whether your glaucoma is well controlled. Although dilating drops cause blurred vision for up to 24 hours, the procedure will not in any way damage your eyes.

4 / Why does my ophthalmologist shine bright lights in my eye at every examination?

In order to diagnose glaucoma your eye specialist needs to examine the optic nerve thoroughly. To do this, he or she needs to shine lights into your eyes. Although the bright lights are uncomfortable they will not permanently affect your vision or damage your eyes.

5 / Is the visual field test bad for my eyes?

No. Although patients are expected to sit for up to twenty minutes concentrating carefully on the visual field target, the test does not cause any damage to the eyes. The test itself may make the eyes feel tired but they soon recover with no permanent long-term effects.

6 / Why must I have a visual field test so often?

The visual field test is an extremely important part of the eye examination for glaucoma. Glaucoma causes loss of side vision long before central vision becomes damaged, and the only way to test side vision is with the visual field test. Although this test is tiring for most patients, the results are very helpful in determining whether your glaucoma is under control. If your ophthalmologist notices a change in your visual field test you will be informed and your treatment will be adjusted accordingly.

7 / Does the field test cause discomfort?

In some patients, yes. Up to 30 per cent of the population experiences difficulty with the test. It requires prolonged concentration without moving the eyes for up to twenty minutes at a time. Many patients find this test tiring. If you need to rest in the middle of the test you should mention this to the technician.

8 / What is a diurnal tension curve?

The diurnal tension curve shows changes in eye pressure. It is well known that intraocular pressure varies throughout the day. This variation is particularly marked in patients with glaucoma. It is possible that you could visit your eye doctor with a normal pressure at 4 p.m. but have a high pressure at 8 a.m. Therefore your eye doctor may ask you to stay a full day at the office and have your pressure checked every hour or two until the office closes. In university hospitals this test can often go on until late at night or early into the following morning. The test is used to determine your pressure profile. Treatment often depends on the results of the whole-day test.

9 / What methods are used to measure pressure?

The most common technique used to measure pressure involves the use of a machine called a Goldmann tonometer. This small device is applied to your eye during a routine eye examination. You may notice a blue light very close to your eye. This blue-light test is used by the eye specialist to check your pressure.

10 / What is the yellow dye placed in my eye before a pressure test?

Fluorescein is a harmless dye that shows bright green in the presence of blue light. The application of fluorescein allows the eye specialist to accurately measure your pressure with the tonometer.

11 / I have undergone a procedure in which I'm told to lie flat while the specialist puts a metal device on my eye. What is the purpose of this?

This is a form of pressure testing called Schiötz tonometry. It is a very old method of pressure testing, and has generally fallen into disuse.

12 / What other methods exist to check pressure?

There are a number of other methods to check pressure, including puff tonometry. A puff tonometer is a device that measures intraocular pressure after delivering a blast of air to the eye. Other pressure testing techniques include one which uses a small computerized pen-like device to measure pressure (tonopen). Other newer tests include dynamic contour tonometry and the ocular response analyser (ORA). The Goldmann blue-light test (see question 9) remains the 'gold standard' for pressure testing.

13 / I recently underwent scanning laser ophthalmoscopy (HRT testing). What is this?

The scanning laser ophthalmoscope is a device that uses a laser beam to scan the optic nerve (see question 17). Studies indicate that this device accurately measures the amount of damage to the optic nerve by measuring the size of the cup and the rim area (see question 15 under All about Glaucoma for further explanation). It is presently believed that the scanning laser ophthalmoscope allows for accurate measurement of early changes in the nerve at the back of the eye and can detect progressive damage before progression is seen by the specialist or detected on the visual field test.

14 / Is the HRT dangerous?

No. The amount of light used during scanning laser ophthalmoscopy is much less than that used in standard eye photography. There is no evidence that HRT (Heidelberg retinal tomography) in any way damages the eye.

15 / What are optic nerve photographs? Why do I need them?

Optic nerve photographs are taken to establish a baseline of optic nerve damage. At subsequent visits your eye doctor will compare the state of your optic nerves with the images on your photos. This will provide information about whether your glaucoma is stable or not.

16 / Will the bright flashes of the photos damage my eyes?

No. Although the bright flashes may cause temporary discomfort, they will not damage your eyes.

17 / What is HRT?

Optic nerve head imaging is available using a special scanning laser ophthalmoscope called a Heidelberg retinal tomograph (HRT). This fast scanner produces a three-dimensional image of the optic nerve. The results from the scan allow specialists to diagnose damage at an early stage. Research has shown that the HRT can also detect early progression of glaucoma caused by nerve damage (see questions 13 and 14).

18 / What is the nerve fibre layer analyser (GDX)?

This is a high-tech imaging device that scans and produces images of the back of the eye. This provides information about the health of the nerve fibre layer that passes to the optic nerve. In glaucoma, the nerve fibre layer thins out. This thinning can be detected using the nerve fibre analyser. This imaging test is used to detect early damage.

19 / What is OCT?

OCT stands for optical coherent tomography. It is an imaging tool that uses a laser beam to visualize structures in the retina. Research shows this technology can be used to detect glaucoma damage that is retinal thinning. This device also has the potential to detect early progression in glaucoma. It is possible that OCT testing could eventually become the major imaging technology for diagnosis and progression analysis in glaucoma. OCT, HRT, and GDX all test for different signs of damage from glaucoma. They can be considered complementary to each other.

20 / What is frequency doubling perimetry?

This is a newer type of visual field test. It is easy to do, fast, and accurate. It is mainly used to screen new patients for glaucoma damage but developments could allow for its use to follow patients who already have glaucoma.

21 / Are there any blood tests for glaucoma?

No, but genetic testing is available for selected types of rare forms of glaucoma (see question 22).

22 / Is there a role for genetic testing in glaucoma?

Genetic tests are available for a minority of selected types of glaucoma. Genetic abnormalities have been detected in some glaucomas including certain types of congenital/developmental glaucoma, juvenile glaucoma, and pigmentary glaucoma. Unfortunately, the majority of glaucoma patients (95 per cent) do not have a genetic abnormality detectable with current genetic tests.

Genetic testing for glaucoma is not simple. It requires highly specialized expertise not available at many medical centres and clinics. However, there is a lot of research interest in genetic testing for glaucoma. If you have a very strong family history of glaucoma developing at a young age (in the 20s or 30s), genetic testing may be right for you. Speak to your glaucoma specialist for advice on genetic testing.

23 / What is corneal thickness testing (pachymetry)?

The thickness of the cornea influences the pressure reading. The thicker the cornea, the higher the reading. The thinner the cornea, the lower the pressure reading. In some people high pressure readings are simply due to the fact that their corneas are excessively thick while in others an eye pressure test registers normal or low due to a thin cornea. It is therefore very important for your doctor to know whether your cornea is normal or excessively thin or thick. Corneal thickness is measured using a pen-like device that is placed on your cornea for a few seconds. This device is called a pachymeter. It measures corneal thickness, most often using ultrasound. Normal corneal thickness is approximately 550 microns. If your reading is 600 microns your true pressure is about 2 points *lower* than the measured result. If your cornea is 500 microns then your true pressure reading is about 2 points *higher* than measured. A thin cornea is a risk factor for glaucoma. Don't forget to ask your eye doctor whether your cornea is of normal thickness.

All about Treatment

Eye Drops

1 / What is target IOP?

Target pressure (IOP) is the pressure reading set by your specialist once glaucoma has been diagnosed. In mild glaucoma and normal pressure glaucoma the target reading is usually set about 30 per cent below a patient's presenting pressure level. In severe disease we aim for a target level about 40 per cent below a patient's presenting pressure level. Target pressures are reset as time goes by according to a patient's treatment response.

2 / What if I forget to take my eye drops?

Take them as soon as you remember. In order to control your glaucoma, drops should be applied regularly, according to your doctor's instructions.

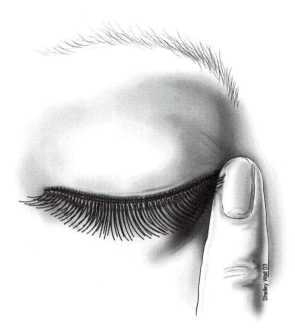

Naso-lacrimal occlusion (see question 3) prevents drops from passing into the nose.

3 / What about side effects from drops? Can they be avoided?

Certain eye drops can adversely affect the lungs and heart in some circumstances (see question 16). To prevent this keep your eyes closed for three minutes after instillation. It is recommended you push on the side of the nose where your upper and lower eyelids meet (applying this pressure is called nasolacrimal occlusion). This prevents drops from entering the nose through the tiny channels that drain tears from the eye. Nasolacrimal occlusion can prevent systemic absorption of drops by up to 40 per cent.

4 / I use three eye drops. How far apart should I space these drops?

It is not advisable to put your drops into your eye all at once. You should wait at least three to five minutes between drops. This prevents dilution and loss of drug in the form of teardrops.

5 / Does it matter which drop goes in first?

If one of the drops you are taking is a long acting Beta blocker like Timoptic-XE®, it should go into your eye last.

6 / Do the eye drops cause cataracts?

Modern-day eye drops may possibly increase the risk of cataracts in some patients. Some of the older eye drops, such as Phospholine Iodide, predisposed patients to cataract formation. Eye doctors therefore tend not to use very strong miotic drops such as Phospholine Iodide (now discontinued) in patients who still have a normal lens.

7 / Can I miss the occasional eye drop?

No. Every time you forget to put an eye drop into your eye there will be no medication in the eye to control the pressure. Consequently, the pressure may increase, causing further damage to your sight. Consistent self-treatment is an essential part of preventing blindness from glaucoma.

8 / How can I prevent contamination when using eye drops?

When applying eye drops, always wash your hands first. Do not touch the dropper tip or let it touch your eye, eyelashes, or any other surface. Why? Because this could contaminate the top with bacteria that may cause eye infection. Always close the bottle when finished and replace the bottle every six weeks.

A / Miotics (Pilocarpine, Isopto® Carpine, Carbachol, Phospholine Iodide®)

9/ How do miotics work?

Miotics, used less commonly these days, lower eye pressure by increasing the flow of fluid out of the drainage system located in the angle of the eye.

10 / If my vision is worse with a miotic drop does this mean I am allergic to this drop?

No. All miotics make the pupil small. This can lead to a decrease in vision because less light is allowed into the eye. This is an unavoidable side effect of miotics. If you experience this side effect, do not stop using your eye drop, but mention the change in your vision to your eye doctor.

11 / If my vision is worse with a miotic should I stop using it?

No. Unfortunately, miotics make your pupil small, which, as indicated above, can lead to a decrease in vision. However, miotics are very effective in lowering pressure in the eye, preventing damage from glaucoma. If your vision is worse with a miotic continue to use the drop and mention this side effect to your eye doctor.

12 / What are the side effects of miotic eye drops?

The common side effects include eye or brow pain, dim vision, blurriness of vision, and occasional redness of the eyes. Fortunately, however, most patients are able to tolerate these side effects. Very occasionally retinal damage may possibly occur. With retinal detachment the patient will typically see flashing lights and small dark floating spots. This may be followed by a curtain-like blocking of the vision.

Patients experiencing these symptoms should stop using the drops and see their eye doctor immediately. Miotic drops are not used as often as they were in the past as a result of the introduction of effective newer drops with fewer side effects (see questions 18 and 27).

13 / Miotics give me a headache. Should I stop using them?

No. Miotics often initially produce severe eye discomfort. However, after a few days the pain settles down and goes away. In a small minority of patients, however, some mild pain continues. If the pain is very severe, simple analgesics usually control it. In most patients the pain will eventually disappear after a few days.

14 / Will I ever be able to stop using my drops?

No. Glaucoma never gets better. You should never stop using your drops unless instructed to do so by your eye doctor.

B / Beta Blockers (Timolol [Timoptic®, Timoptic-XE®], Levobunolol [Betagan®], Betaxolol [Betoptic S®])

15 / I use a beta blocker. What are they and how do they work?

These drugs inhibit the formation of eye fluid. This decreased production leads to lower intraocular pressure. There are many types of beta blocker eye drops. They all work in a similar fashion by reducing the flow of the aqueous fluid into the eye. Examples of beta blockers are Timolol, Levobunolol, and Betaxolol. Most are used twice a day. Timoptic-XE® and its generic forms are made from a thick gel and are used once a day, usually first thing in the morning.

16 / I have asthma. Can I use beta blockers?

No. Beta blocker eye drops should not be used by patients with asthma as they can aggravate this condition. Betaxolol has less effect on lung function than do other beta blockers, but it too can occasionally affect lung function, especially in asthmatics.

17 / Do beta blockers produce any side effects?

Beta blockers such as Timolol usually produce few side effects. However, patients with asthma and heart failure or heart block can find that these conditions are made worse by this group of drugs. On rare occasions beta blockers produce psychological problems such as depression, sleep disturbances, and impotence. Cold fingers and poor circulation are sometimes a problem. Blood cholesterol levels can be increased by some beta blockers. Betaxolol (Betoptic S®) produces fewer heart and lung problems.

C / Adrenergic Agents (Brimonidine, Iopidine)

18 / What is Alphagan™/Alphagan P®?

Alphagan™ (brimonidine) is used to treat open-angle glaucoma and ocular hypertension. It works mainly by lowering the production of fluid in the eye. Alphagan P® has a slightly lower concentration of active drug than Alphagan™ and has a different preservative. Alphagan P® produces fewer side effects than Alphagan.

19 / How do I use Alphagan™/Alphagan P® eye drops?

One drop of brimonidine should be dropped into the affected eye usually twice daily – each dose taken 12 hours apart. It can be used three times a day if directed by your doctor. If you miss your dose, apply the drops as soon as you remember. If you wear contact lenses, they should be removed before you apply the drops. You can put back your contacts after 15 minutes.

20 / What are some of the side effects of Alphagan™ or Alphagan P®?

A fairly large number of people experience an allergic reaction, namely red, irritable, and itchy eyes, with this drop. Occasionally, some people may experience drowsiness and

fatigue when using Alphagan™. Alphagan P®
produces fewer allergic reactions than Alpha-
gan™. Other side effects include whitening
of the eye followed hours later by redness,
dry mouth, burning/stinging of the eyes,
blurred vision, dizziness, and headaches. See
your doctor if any of these symptoms persist.
Alphagan™ and Alphagan P® should never be
given to infants.

21 / What are the side effects of other adrenergic agonist eye drops?

Epinephrine-like eye drops are no longer
widely used to treat glaucoma. However,
when used they often cause the eye to become red with a slightly dilated pupil. More
unusual side effects include raised blood pressure, angina, and excessive sweating.

22 / Do these drugs cause allergic reactions?

Allergic responses are common with Alpha-
gan™ drops. Often they initially cause the eye
to become whiter than usual, and then red a
few hours after instillation. Other side effects
include dilated pupils and rapid heart rate.

23 / What is Apraclonidine (Iopidine®)?

Iopidine® is used to prevent pressure increases
after laser treatment. A drop of Iopidine®

is inserted in the eye one hour before and one hour after laser treatment. The drop significantly prevents pressure spikes – large, sudden increases in pressure – in patients needing glaucoma laser surgery. Long term use is curtailed by side effects.

24 / What are the side effects from Iopidine®?

Iopidine® commonly causes irritation and redness of the eye and allergic reactions. It can also produce nasal discomfort. Its effectiveness decreases over time in some patients. For these reasons it is not prescribed for the long term.

D / Topical Carbonic Anhydrase Inhibitors (Trusopt®/Azopt™)

25 / What is Dorzolamide (Trusopt®)?

Dorzolamide (Trusopt®) is a carbonic anhydrase inhibitor. It is applied in drop form to the eye usually two or three times per day. It does not cause many of the side effects associated with oral administration of these drugs (see question 41). This drug effectively lowers intraocular pressure, both when used alone or in combination with other eye drops. It should not be used in patients with a known sulfonamide allergy. In theory it can result in failure of blood cells to mature (a condition known as aplastic anemia) but this has not been proven to date.

This drop often stings when it is inserted, and it can produce an unpleasant taste in the mouth. An allergic reaction causing a red itchy eye or lid can also occur.

26 / What is Brinzolamide (Azopt™)?

Brinzolamide (Azopt™) is similar to Dorzol-amide. It belongs to the class of medications called topical carbonic anhydrase inhibitors and is associated with sulfonamides. It helps lower the pressure in the eye by reducing inflow of eye fluid. Its effects on eye pressure are similar to Trusopt® (dorzolamide) but it tends to produce less stinging. As it is a sus-pension it can cause accumulation of white matter on the lashes, resulting in the need for regular eyelash cleaning.

E / Topical Prostaglandin Agents (Xalatan™/Lumigan®/Travatan® Z)

27 / What is Xalatan™?

Xalatan™ (latanoprost) is a potent prescrip-tion eyedrop used to treat glaucoma. It is part of a family of medications called prostaglan-din analogues. It helps lower the pressure in the eye by increasing the outflow of fluid from inside the eye.

28 / How are Xalatan™ eye drops used?

One drop of Xalatan™ should be dropped into the affected eye once daily. It is recommended that you do this at the same time every night before bed time. If you wear contact lenses, they should be removed before you use Xalatan™. Your contacts can be put back in 15 minutes after using the eye drops.

29 / What are some of the side effects of Xalatan™?

Some patients using Xalatan™ may notice a gradual change in eye colour, but it may go unnoticed for months or even years. Xalatan™ can increase the amount of brown pigment in the iris (the coloured part of the eye) and this effect is more apparent in people with eye colours such as blue/gray or green/brown. If you experience changes in eye colour, your doctor can stop treatment but any colour change that occurs is permanent. Xalatan™ can also cause your eyelashes to darken, thicken, and grow longer than normal. Sometimes fine hair can be found growing below the lid and lid darkening may occur. Xalatan™ can also cause eye irritation. It may possibly produce inflammation in the eye (iritis) or cause vision to decrease from retinal swelling, but this side effect is rare. The drops may occasionally reactivate a viral infection in a previously infected, predisposed eye (Herpes Simplex virus). Finally, your eyes may also become red and watery.

30 / What are Lumigan® and Lumigan® RC (Bimatoprost)?

Lumigan®, like Travatan® and Xalatan™, belongs to the prostaglandin family of drugs. It is an effective pressure-lowering drop. Like Travatan® and Xalatan™, this drop is used once a day (usually at the same time every night) to lower eye pressure. Its use can be associated with red eyes, which may improve somewhat with continued use of the drop. The RC version (reduced concentration) has fewer side effects. Some patients resistant to Xalatan™ can experience pressure reduction with this drop. It has similar side effects to Travatan® and Xalatan™ (see questions 31 and 29).

31 / What is Travatan® Z (Travoprost)?

Travatan® Z, like Lumigan® and Xalatan™, is a prostaglandin drop used to effectively lower eye pressure. Like Xalatan™ and Lumigan®, it can cause red eyes, which may improve somewhat with continued use of the drop. This drop may reduce pressure in some patients who do not respond to Xalatan™. Its side effects are similar to those of Lumigan® and Xalatan™ (see questions 29 and 30).

32 / What is Tafluprost (Taflotan®)?

This drug is also a prostaglandin agent but is the only one in this class without preservative. As preservatives in drops irritate the eye this drug is of value for patients with preservative allergy. It isn't available as yet in North America but is available in the UK and Europe.

F / *Combination Drops*

33 / What is Cosopt®?

Cosopt® is a prescription medication for the treatment of elevated intraocular pressure in patients with ocular hypertension, open-angle, and closed-angle glaucoma. It is made up of two commonly used drugs called timolol maleate (Timoptic®) and dorzolamide hydrochloride (Trusopt®) (see above questions 15 and 25). Both of these drugs lower intraocular pressure. When they are combined, the effect is greater than using one or the other alone. Cosopt® offers the strength of two medications without the bother of taking two separate drugs. This makes it more convenient for patients who need to take more than one medication to control intraocular pressure. A preservative-free version of this drop is available for patients with preservative allergy.

34 / What are some of the side effects of Cosopt®?

You may experience some eye symptoms such as burning and stinging, redness of the eye, tearing, itching, and blurred vision. Other possible side effects include dizziness, nausea, headache, drowsiness, loss of appetite, bitter taste in the mouth, tiredness (very occasionally), loss of weight, stomach upset, and depression. If such symptoms occur and persist, see your eye doctor for advice. Cosopt® should not be used in patients with known asthma, heart failure, or heart block.

35 / What is Xalacom™ (Xalatan™/Timolol maleate combination)?

Xalacom™ is a combination eye drop made from a prostaglandin agent and a beta-blocker (Xalatan™ and Timolol). It is used once a day. This combination eye drop had been shown to work better than Xalatan™ or Timolol alone, but interestingly, it may not work quite as well as the two individual drops when both are used separately. It is important to know that Xalacom™ has the same side effects as the prostaglandins and the beta-blockers (see questions 17 and 29). Before use ask your glaucoma doctor about the possible side effects of this combination drop.

36 / What is Combigan® (Timolol maleate/ Alphagan™)?

This is a combination drop, used every 12 hours, made from Timolol and Alphagan™ (see questions 15 and 18). Before use ask your doctor about the possible side effects of this drop. See also questions 17 and 20 for details regarding possible side effects.

37 / What is Ganfort® (Timolol/Lumigan™)?

This combination drop is not currently available in Canada. It is made from Timolol and Lumigan®. Please see relevant questions 17 and 30 above for side effects from each part of this drop.

38 / What is DuoTrav®?

This is a combination of Timolol maleate and Travatan® (see questions 15 and 31).

39 / What is Azarga®?

This is a combination of Timolol maleate and Azopt® (see questions 15 and 26).

Oral Medications

40 / Can tablets such as Diamox® and Neptazane® help treat my glaucoma, and if so, how?

Tablets are sometimes useful in treating glaucoma. Acetazolamide and Methazolamide

(Diamox® and Neptazane®) are prescribed for glaucoma. They effectively lower the pressure in the eye by decreasing the amount of eye fluid produced. Methazolamide is no longer available in some countries.

41 / Do tablets such as Diamox® or Neptazane® have any side effects?

As with any medication, these tablets can produce side effects. Common problems include tingling in the fingers and toes, frequent urination, stomach upset, weight loss, feelings of depression or tiredness, formation of kidney stones, and, very occasionally, failure of the blood cells to mature (called aplastic anemia), a condition which can be fatal. Luckily, however, this last side effect is extremely rare. Potassium loss can be a problem when these tablets are taken at the same time as thiazide diuretics (used to treat high blood pressure). These drugs should not be taken by patients using digoxin, ciprofloxacin, aspirin, and methenamine. Patients with gout should not take these drugs. To prevent problems, it is critical that you tell your doctor about all the medications you are taking. It is also probably advisable to occasionally have your family doctor check your electrolytes and blood count if you are taking these medications.

Other Medications

42 / Is smoking marijuana beneficial in glaucoma?

Intraocular pressure can be lowered by smoking marijuana. However, the effect is not long lasting. A person with glaucoma would have to smoke a marijuana cigarette every two hours – about 4000 a year – to experience a sustained pressure-lowering effect. In view of the fact that marijuana's effect on intraocular pressure is not prolonged, it should not be used to treat glaucoma. There are much better eye drop medications currently available for glaucoma therapy.

Patient Compliance

43 / Is there anything I can do to prevent vision loss?

You can help preserve your vision by taking your glaucoma treatment (eye drops) exactly as prescribed by your doctor. Many people miss their doses for a variety of reasons such as forgetfulness, inconvenience, or side effects. It is important to get into a routine to ensure you do not forget to take the drops. Remember to wait about 5 minutes between drops.

44 / I often forget to take my medications. What can I do to improve this?

Many glaucoma medications need to be taken

more than once a day, and for this reason patients often have problems following the dosing schedule. Taking your medications exactly as prescribed is very important in the proper treatment of glaucoma. Missing doses because it's inconvenient or you forget can lead to an increase in pressure, and that can eventually lead to vision loss. You should mention this issue to your doctor, especially if the drops are not being used as directed. Ask your doctor about devices or treatment options, including non-drop options such as laser treatment or surgery, that may be more convenient for your specific situation. As a way to remind you to take the drops, consider buying an alarm watch or use a cell phone alarm to remind you when to insert your drops. Check-off sheets or a diary can help remind you to take your drops.

45 / How do I put in eye drops?

Wash your hands, then tilt your head back and look at the ceiling. Use your index finger from one hand to pull down your lower eye lid to create a pocket. Squeeze one drop into the pocket, close the eye for a minute and dab the excess away with a wet cloth. Wait 3 to 5 minutes before inserting the next drop into this eye. Please visit http://www.nyee.edu/video-ritch-sussman.html to learn how to instill your drops.

Laser Treatment

1 / What is laser trabeculoplasty?

Laser trabeculoplasty is the standard laser procedure performed on patients with chronic open-angle glaucoma. A laser beam is applied to the trabecular meshwork (the drainage portion located in the angle of the eye), usually in two sessions approximately one to two months apart (see figure 4, p. 80). The procedure is done while the patient is sitting at the slit lamp. It is painless, performed without a need for anaesthesia. It does, however, cause the patient to see bright flashes of light, and some patients complain of mild discomfort during the procedure.

2 / What is selective laser trabeculoplasty (SLT)?

Selective laser trabeculoplasty uses a special wavelength of laser light to more accurately focus the treating laser light on the cells in the drainage system. Although this form of laser treatment does not produce better pressure lowering than Argon laser treatment, it has the theoretical advantage of causing less long-term damage to the drainage system, and seems to allow for more than the usual two treatments.

3 / Does laser treatment cause cataracts?

There is no evidence that laser treatment causes cataracts.

4 / Will laser treatment cure my glaucoma?

Laser trabeculoplasty will not cure your glaucoma. In most cases it brings the eye pressure back under control by improving drainage of fluid from the eye. Fifty per cent of cases treated in this manner are still controlled five years after the procedure.

5 / What are the dangers of laser trabeculoplasty?

Laser trabeculoplasty is remarkably safe. Although many people think laser treatment makes holes in the drainage system of the eye, it does not. The laser supplies energy to the cells lining the drainage system, producing complex chemical and biomechanical reactions leading to improved drainage through the drainage system. However, eye pressure can sometimes increase suddenly after treatment. This increase in pressure can be controlled with appropriate medications. Your eye specialist will usually ask you to stay at the office for at least an hour after the procedure to ensure that your pressure has not jumped to unacceptable levels. Other minor complications include mild visual disturbance for a few hours, and a slightly inflamed eye for a few days.

6 / Does Argon or selective laser trabeculoplasty always work?

No. Laser trabeculoplasty has a high success rate during the first year after treatment.

However, by the five-year mark only about 50 per cent of patients still have well-controlled pressures.

7 / Do I need to continue using my drops after laser treatment?

Yes. After laser treatment patients are not usually able to stop using their eye drops. Laser therapy does, however, bring the uncontrolled pressure back within normal limits in patients on eye-drop treatment.

8 / Can laser treatment be used alone?

Yes. Patients who are allergic to or intolerant of drops or tablets can undergo laser treatment as a primary form of therapy.

9 / Why do I need laser treatment if my vision is good?

It is critical to understand that with glaucoma, central vision is not affected until very late in the disease.

10 / What is a laser iridotomy?

A laser iridotomy is a hole made in the coloured part of the eye (the iris). It is done to treat acute glaucoma or to prevent acute glaucoma from developing (see question 24 under All about Glaucoma). It is also used to treat patients with some other forms of angle-closure glaucoma (see figure 3).

11 / Can laser iridotomy result in a hole that is too large? What are the other complications?

Laser iridotomy usually produces a very small hole. Occasionally the hole does allow extra light into the eye, resulting in the patient seeing a horizontal, slightly discolored line that appears to move with blinking. This visual disturbance is not serious at all and will not affect vision. Usually simple reassurance is all that is required to alleviate the symptom. Other very rare complications of laser treatment include damage to the lens, retina, or cornea. Other complications include transient pressure spikes, bleeding from the iris, and mild inflammation of the eye. These latter three complications respond well to appropriate therapy and cause no long-term problems.

12 / How long should I stay home from work after laser treatment?

Laser treatment (both iridotomy and trabeculoplasty) should not affect your ability to work. Usually you can go back to work the day after the procedure. Very occasionally, laser treatment can produce inflammation, which may make the eye uncomfortable. In this situation you may have to stay home from work for a couple of days.

13 / I have been told I need a ciliary body destructive procedure. What is this?

Destruction of the ciliary body (a procedure called cycloablation) is done either with a laser beam, or with a cryoprobe (a freezing device). It is a treatment used on eyes where conventional treatment is unlikely to work. Transscleral diode cyclocoagulation (done with a laser) is currently the procedure of choice to treat patients with severe glaucoma. The procedure is done under local anaesthetic. It takes approximately ten minutes, and has a success rate of approximately 60 per cent. Complications include loss of vision in about 10 per cent of cases, pain and discomfort, a red eye for a few weeks, and excessively low pressure. In view of these complications this procedure is performed only in cases where blindness is a significant risk. Freezing treatment (cyclocryotherapy) achieves similar results but is associated with more complications, and is therefore used less often than laser treatment. It is most commonly used on blind, painful eyes with high pressure, but can be very effective in select cases.

14 / What is direct ciliary process laser treatment (endocyclophotocoagulation)?

The ciliary processes (the tissue producing the eye fluid) can be examined by an eye surgeon and destroyed using a laser beam. Unlike the usual ciliary body destructive procedure known as transscleral diode cyclo-photocoagulation (see question 13), this form of surgery requires direct entry into the eye during eye surgery so the surgeon can focus the laser beam onto the ciliary processes. As this requires opening the eye and is a major surgical procedure it is sometimes done in conjunction with cataract surgery. Complications from this form of surgery are similar to those described in question 13, and added to these are the risks associated with opening the eyeball to allow the surgeon access to the ciliary processes.

Surgery

1 / What kind of surgical treatment is available for glaucoma? How successful is it?

Filtration surgery, which creates a new drainage system from within the eye to under the lining membrane of the eye (conjunctiva), is called trabeculectomy (see figures 5 and 6, pp. 81 and 82). The surgery is done under local anaesthesia and takes about three-quarters of an hour to perform. It is done using an operating microscope. This surgery has a success rate of approximately 75–90 per cent. Some people, however, do need to continue to use eye drops after surgery. Unfortunately, approximately 10 per cent of patients require more than one operation to bring the pressure under control. Very occasionally, the surgery can actually cause vision loss, but this occurs in less than 5 per cent of patients.

2 / Does glaucoma surgery cause cataracts?

There is some evidence to suggest that patients who undergo glaucoma surgery may have an increased tendency to form cataracts. As previously discussed, loss of sight from cataracts can be surgically treated. Loss of sight from glaucoma, however, is irreversible.

3 / Do I need to stay in hospital if I have glaucoma surgery?

In North America, patients are usually treated as outpatients; that is, their surgery is done under local anesthetic and they are allowed to go home a few hours later. Patients are, of course, advised to go straight to bed and not to bend over or physically exert themselves for at least forty-eight hours.

4 / Is surgery painful?

Most surgeries are performed under local anaesthetic. This means that you will be awake and you will feel a few pinpricks at the start of the operation. During the operation you will feel pulling sensations but no pain.

You can talk to your surgeon if required, but silence is generally preferred.

5 / What happens if I attempt to blink during surgery?

You may feel the need to blink during surgery. A special lid instrument called a speculum will be placed between your eyelids to ensure that they remain open during the whole procedure. Blinking will therefore in no way affect your surgery.

6 / What happens if I cough during surgery?

Slight movements and gentle coughs are not usually a problem during surgery. Severe coughing, however, can be disruptive to the surgeon and make surgery difficult to perform.

7 / Can I see during the operation?

The eye not being operated on will be covered during the surgery. The eye being operated on will be prepared and cleaned with antiseptic, and then the local anesthetic will be administered. Some local anesthetics cause loss of vision while others do not. Ask your surgeon which type of local anesthetic is to be used in your case. If it is the latter, you will see a bright light with moving shadows during the operation.

8 / Will my eye hurt after surgery?

Once the local anesthetic wears off you may feel some pain, especially when moving the eye or blinking. If this occurs simply keep both eyelids closed and take a painkiller. Most patients do not need one, but do check with your family practitioner before surgery regarding the appropriate painkiller for you. Severe eye pain is most unusual after glaucoma surgery; if you do experience severe pain you should contact your eye surgeon for further advice.

9 / What can go wrong during eye surgery?

Trabeculectomy has been the standard operation for glaucoma for over forty years, and it is generally a safe, effective procedure. However, complications occasionally occur. They can include injury from the local anesthetic injection (very rare) and intraocular bleeding. Mild bleeding is usually not a problem for the patient or surgeon. It can, however, lead to prolonged rehabilitation. Sudden bursting of a blood vessel in the eye during or after surgery causes severe pain and is an extremely rare complication that can lead to permanent vision loss. Other surgical difficulties can and do occasionally occur. Usually they can all be dealt with by a competent surgeon, but some complications may result in a prolonged recovery.

10 / What are antifibroblastic agents?

Antifibroblastic agents are drugs that are used to prevent healing of the surgical wound, and thereby improve the chances of successful surgery. They are used on patients requiring repeat surgery or who have complicated glaucomas. There are two drugs in this family:

*5-Fluorouracil (5-FU).*This anticancer drug effectively improves surgical success, especially in patients who have previously had unsuccessful surgery, or in patients who have previously had cataract surgery. The drug can be applied during surgery, or administered daily via injections to the surface of the eye for a period of three to five days. Complications from the drug include corneal ulcers and eye discomfort. Corneal ulcers sometimes develop on the front of the eye after four or more treatments. These ulcers can be painful but usually settle down within a few weeks after treatment with drops and the wearing of an eye patch.

Mitomycin. This anticancer drug is an effective antihealing agent. It is applied during surgery to the surgical site. It is more convenient for both patient and surgeon than 5-FU because of its intraoperative use. Complications, however, can be more serious than with 5-FU. This drug is so effective that it can produce excessive drainage of fluid through the newly created surgical site. The low pressure that can result is known as hypotony and can be associated with a larger than usual bleb (see question 23) and a soft eye. A soft eye, that is, one with pressure below 6 mmHg, may result in decreased vision. If the eye remains excessively soft over a long period of time it can be treated with injections of blood into the wound area, or can be surgically repaired. A large thin bleb can occasionally leak, necessitating antibiotic therapy and surgical repair.

11 / Is there a role for early surgery in glaucoma?

There is a trend towards earlier surgery. There are of course complications associated with surgery, and as a consequence ophthalmic surgeons in North America still recommend drops or laser treatment first and surgery as a last resort.

12 / What is successful surgery?

Surgery is successful when the pressure in the eye is reduced by about 30 per cent, whether the patient is on or off medication. The key to success is a reduction in pressure to a level that prevents ongoing nerve and visual field damage.

13 / What can go wrong after surgery?

Although the success rate for surgery is high (75–90 per cent), complications occasionally occur. These include:

1) Postoperative complications such as a soft eye (called a flat anterior chamber) due to excessive drainage of fluid from the eye (see question 19). This usually heals with appropriate care in five to seven days but does occasionally require surgical intervention to remedy the excessive drainage.
2) Blurred vision for up to six weeks.
3) In rare instances, total loss of vision. It is not clearly understood why this occurs but it does occur in patients with very severe vision loss before the glaucoma surgery.

Other complications include infection, hemorrhaging, damage to the eye or the optic nerve from the local anesthetic injection, discomfort, change in refraction (strength of glasses), droopy lid, and development of ciliary block glaucoma (see question 22).

14 / How will my eye look after surgery?

Immediately after surgery your eye will be bloodshot and swollen. However, over a four- to six-week period it will whiten and should eventually look virtually normal. Occasionally, however, the eyelid may droop a little or you may see a white blob appear from under the upper lid (see question 23).

15 / My eye feels dry after surgery. Is this normal?

It is not uncommon for a patient's eye to feel gritty and dry after surgery. This is usually because the tear film is not spread evenly over the front of the eye. Should this occur it is important to avoid dry environments like air-conditioned cars. Topical lubricants can often relieve this symptom.

16 / My eye feels wet since surgery. Is this normal?

Occasionally after surgery the wound may leak for a few weeks. This usually causes slight dampness, particularly during the night and on awakening. This symptom should be reported to your eye surgeon. There are a number of ways to cure such leaks, including the use of eye patches, topical drops, a contact lens, and, occasionally, surgical repair of the leak. Leaks usually resolve spontaneously.

17 / The doctor massaged my eye after surgery. Is this a routine procedure?

It is common for the eye surgeon to massage the eye after surgery. The purpose of this procedure is to push fluid through the passageway created during the operation. In fact, your eye surgeon may teach you how to massage your own eye. The massage keeps the surgical wound open, keeping the pressure in the eye low. Do not massage your eye unless instructed by your eye surgeon. Initially massage may be uncomfortable, especially if done a day or two after surgery. However, it will not damage the eye if performed by an eye surgeon, or by yourself as directed by your surgeon.

18 / Can high pressure develop after surgery?

High eye pressure after surgery usually means that the new surgical passage is blocked. This can be dealt with by eye massage (see question 17) and by using a laser on stitches (suture lysis) (see question 20).

19 / Can surgery produce a soft eye?

The purpose of the surgery is to allow eye fluid (the aqueous humor) to leave the eye through a covered hole (2 mm × 2 mm) created by your surgeon. On occasion excessive leakage can occur during the early post-operative period. This can lead to a soft eye with a flat anterior chamber. Your surgeon will determine the extent of the over filtration and may recommend the following:

(a) An eye patch. A simple eye patch or protective shield plus drops usually resolves the problem in three to ten days.

(b) Glue or a contact lens over the leaky area,

with or without a patch. In addition, eye
drops are prescribed.

(c) Surgical repair. If the drainage is excessive
it may be necessary to insert air or fluid
into the eye to 'pump up' the eye a little.
Occasionally choroidals are drained after
surgery to help re-form the eye. Choroidals are fluid-filled cyst-like areas that
develop in the eye when the pressure is
very low. Sometimes surgeons place an
extra stitch or two into the surface of
the eye (conjunctiva or sclera) to reduce
the fluid outflow.

20 / My surgeon says I need a suture cut after glaucoma surgery. Is this necessary?

After surgery you may need to have a stitch
cut to help bring the pressure under control.
Cutting a suture is painless for the patient
and easy to do with the laser. It does not require a scalpel blade. It is usually done under
topical anesthesia, that is, with the use of an
eye drop and a special contact lens. The procedure usually takes no more than a couple
of minutes. It is commonly followed by eye
massage (see question 17).

21 / Can surgery cause blindness?

Glaucoma surgery is usually very successful
(see question 1). It is possible, however, that
some patients may lose vision after surgery.

This is extremely rare and usually occurs only in patients with very severe glaucomatous damage at the time of surgery.

22 / My doctor says I have malignant glaucoma (ciliary block). What is this?

Ciliary block glaucoma can develop after surgery, and is characterized by high pressure. The cause of this pressure is a fluid imbalance between the back and the front of the eye. In this condition the fluid passes towards the back of the eye instead of through the normal chambers in the front of the eye. It is called malignant glaucoma by some doctors. This complication has absolutely nothing to do with cancer. The condition is reversible, with the use of eye drops and oral medications, in 50 per cent of the cases. The other 50 per cent require further surgery to remedy the condition.

23 / Since surgery I have noticed a raised white blob under my upper lid. What causes this?

After glaucoma surgery, fluid flows out of the eye under a thin membrane called the conjunctiva. When this membrane swells and is filled with fluid it produces a small balloon-like structure under the upper eyelid called a bleb, which can be seen by lifting the upper lid. It is not a cause for concern. In fact, it is a good sign, as it means the operation has been effective (see figure 6).

24 / Do blebs become less effective with time?

Blebs do shrink with time and can scar up. When this happens, the pressure will increase, eventually leading to the reintroduction of the use of eye drops, and possibly repeat surgery.

25 / Can blebs cause problems?

Large blebs in themselves can produce a number of symptoms including discomfort and irritation. Large blebs can and do push on the eye and cause astigmatism. A change in eyeglass prescription may therefore be required after surgery.

26 / Can blebs cause discomfort?

A dry area occasionally develops in front of the bleb, causing discomfort and some pain. This is readily relieved by using artificial tears to wet the dry area.

27 / My bleb is still present but my pressure is increasing. Is this a problem?

Blebs do become less effective with time for two reasons:

(1) glaucoma often gets worse with age;

(2) blebs tend to scar.

If your pressure starts increasing the ophthalmologist will initially recommend restarting medical therapy, which usually controls the situation. If not, repeat surgery is always an option.

28 / Can blebs have serious complications?

Yes. Blebs very occasionally become infected and/or leak spontaneously. Leaks can occur after excessive trauma to the eye. Leaks can cause low pressure, resulting in blurry vision, and can make the eye susceptible to infection. Infection can be caused by swimming in contaminated water, or from poor lid hygiene. Swimming should be avoided after trabeculectomy surgery. Infections are extremely rare but serious.

29 / How are bleb leaks treated?

The best way to treat bleb leaks is to surgically remove the leaking bleb and replace it with healthy transplanted tissue from elsewhere on the eye. Sometimes a flap of conjunctiva can be transferred or pulled from above to cover the leak. Other less successful but more conservative techniques used to treat bleb leaks include lowering pressure with drops to reduce the flow of fluid through the leak, injecting the area around the leak with blood to block the leak with blood products, contact lenses, eye patching, or glue. These conservative techniques often don't work. The downside to surgery for a leak includes scarring of the transplanted or pulled-down conjunctiva, which in turn can lead to a return of the high eye pressure, necessitating glaucoma drops or more glaucoma surgery.

30 / How do I know if my bleb is infected?

A bleb infection is characterized by a mild to moderate discomfort, a yellow or green discharge, a very red eye, blurry vision, and a white bleb. This is an emergency requiring intensive treatment with antibiotics to prevent loss of vision. If the infection is caught early the eye can often be saved. The bleb, however, may scar or leak after an infection.

31 / Should I take any precautions after my surgery?

Glaucoma surgery is based on the principle of making a new drainage system in the eye. Any excessive exercise or trauma for the first weeks can lead to too much softening of the eye. It is important not to exert oneself excessively for the first two to three weeks following surgery. Sexual activity is permissible after this time period.

32 / My doctor says I need a Molteno/ Ahmed/Baerveldt glaucoma drainage device implant. What is this?

Implants are plastic tube-like devices (called Setons) inserted into the eye to help drainage of fluid from the eye to the tissues surrounding the eye (see front cover picture and figure 7, p. 83). A Seton implant is performed when conventional surgery has failed or as a primary procedure in special situations. The tube bypasses the scarred part of the eye, causing the pressure to come under control. Technically this is a more involved operation than a simple trabeculectomy. Successful control of pressure is often possible. Complications include damage to the cornea, erosion of the tube, high intraocular pressure postoperatively, low intraocular pressure postoperatively, damage to the lens, pain and discomfort for the patient, and double vision. Despite these complications, the success rate for such implants is good. Furthermore, they can save sight in eyes that might otherwise be doomed to blindness.

33 / Are there any other forms of glaucoma surgery? What is canaloplasty?

A newer form of surgery has been developed called non-penetrating surgery. This technique is a modification of the standard procedure. The surgeon does not actually enter the eye but creates a very thin membrane between the inner part of the eye and its surface, allowing the eye fluid to gently pass through the membrane. The surgery is done under a small flap and often a piece of plastic is left under the flap (called a wick) to prevent the wound from closing. A recent modification is called canaloplasty, where the drainage system is dilated and a suture placed in the drain which is then tightened to stretch the outflow system. None of these techniques are widely used in North America as the results indicate that these surgeries do not lower pressure as well as traditional surgery (trabeculectomy – see question 1). The major advantages of these newer surgeries are that they involve faster recovery and fewer complications. You should ask your eye surgeon whether this form of surgery is advisable for you.

34 / What is the trabectome?

The trabectome is a newer surgical device designed to open the drainage channels to allow fluid to leave the eye. It uses an electric current to cauterize the drainage system. The procedure is done in the operating room under local anesthesia. Trabectome surgery, like canaloplasty, doesn't lower pressure as well as trabeculectomy, but it does have fewer complications and faster recovery. Bleeding is expected with the procedure but this usually resolves with appropriate eye drops. A transient pressure increase can occur with this procedure. As the pressure reduction is not as good as traditional surgery this procedure is not the treatment of choice in severe glaucoma. Ask your glaucoma specialist if this is the right procedure for your eye.

35 / What is the ExPress shunt?

The ExPress shunt is a modification of trabeculectomy surgery. The difference however is that a small stainless steel shunt is placed into the eye to create the drainage channel. The procedure has certain advantages including faster surgery and less post-operative inflammation. It is more expensive surgery as a metal device is used. Early results suggest that this shunt provides good pressure control, equal to trabeculectomy. It is possible this procedure could one day challenge trabeculectomy as the procedure of choice.

36 / What other surgical procedures exist for glaucoma?

There are a number of other experimental procedures undergoing trial for glaucoma, including evaluation of the iStent. The results are possibly similar to the trabectome and canaloplasty but not as good as trabeculectomy or ExPress shunt. Time will tell if such surgeries have a place in routine surgical care for glaucoma patients.

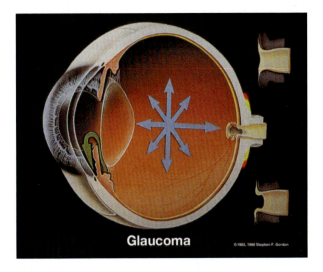

Glaucoma

©1983, 1989 Stephen F. Gordon

Figure 1: Flow of fluid through the eye. Obstruction to flow in the front of the eye (green arrows) increases pressure in the eye (blue arrows) leading to damage to the optic nerve at the back of the eye. The depressed area in the middle of the optic nerve is the result of an abnormal process called cupping.

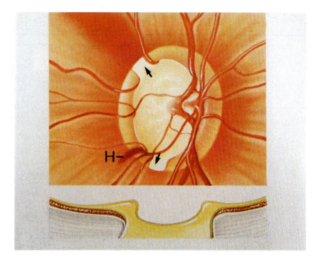

Figure 2: Nerve damage in glaucoma. The central white area is known as the cup. The arrows show areas of damage (notches) on the rim of the nerve. 'H' is a hemorrhage on the rim of the nerve. Hemorrhages, notches, and cupping occur if the pressure in the eye is at an unacceptable level. The bottom of the picture shows a severely cupped nerve.

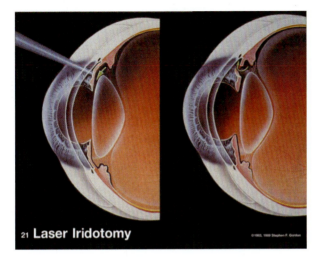

21 Laser Iridotomy

© 1993, 1999 Stephen F. Gordon

Figure 3: Effect of a laser burn (iridotomy) on the iris to treat or prevent acute glaucoma. The arrow shows the unimpeded passage of fluid through the hole created by the laser burn.

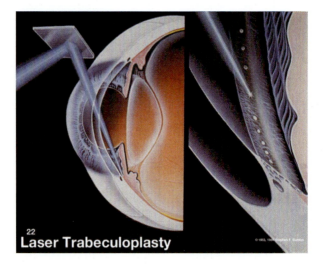

Figure 4: Laser trabeculoplasty. The laser is focused through a mirror into the trabecular meshwork in the angle of the eye. The white spots show the heating effect caused by the laser.

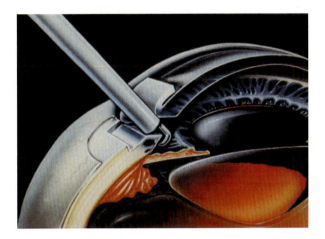

Figure 5: Filtration surgery. Note the creation of a
channel to allow the fluid to leave the eye.

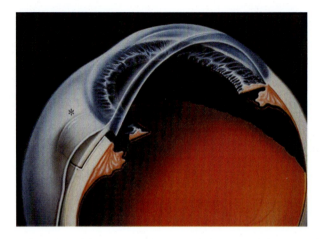

Figure 6: This shows the end result of a trabeculectomy surgical procedure. A trap door covered by a membrane called a bleb (see asterisk) allows the fluid to leave the eye.

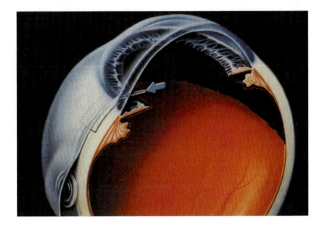

Figure 7: A glaucoma drainage device. The blue arrow indicates the passage of fluid from inside the eye through the tube to a base plate well away from the scarred surgical site.

Glaucoma Societies

1 / In Canada

The Glaucoma Research Society of Canada is an organization run by members of the public that depends on charitable donations to help fund research at academic institutions. Dr Trope is the founder member and Scientific Advisory Board director of this charity. Their address is:

Glaucoma Research Society of Canada
1929 Bayview Avenue, Suite 215E
Toronto, Ontario, M4G 3E8
(416) 260-4267, fax (416) 204-1939.
http://www.glaucomaresearch.ca

2 / In the United States

The Glaucoma Research Foundation supports glaucoma research.
251 Post St., Ste 600
San Francisco, CA 94108
(415) 986-3162, fax (415) 986-3763
www.glaucoma.org

The Glaucoma Foundation
80 Maiden Lane, Suite 700
New York, NY 10038 USA
Tel: 212-651-1900
Fax: 212-651-1888
e-mail: scott@glaucomafoundation.org
Website: www.glaucomafoundation.org

3 / In the United Kingdom
International Glaucoma Association:
www.glaucoma-association.com

Other Reference Materials

http://www.nyee.edu/video-ritch-sussman.html.
This video shows you how to put in eye drops.

Coping with Glaucoma
By Edith Marks, Avery Publishing Group, New
York.

Glossary of Glaucoma Terms

adrenergic agents. A class of eye drops that reduces eye pressure mainly by decreasing production and increasing outflow of aqueous humour.

angle-closure glaucoma. An unusual and painful form of glaucoma requiring emergency medical and laser treatment.

antifibroblastic agents. Anticancer drugs used to prevent scarring after glaucoma surgery.

aplastic anemia. A potentially lethal form of blood thinning occasionally caused by carbonic anhydrase inhibitors.

aqueous humour. The interior eye fluid produced by the ciliary processes. This fluid nourishes the front of the eye and drains out through the trabecular mesh-work. Eye pressure is modified by changes in production or drainage of this fluid.

beta blockers. The most commonly used class of glaucoma eye drops. Beta blockers inhibit the formation of aqueous humour, thereby lowering intraocular pressure. They can precipitate asthma and heart failure in susceptible individuals.

bleb. A raised swelling usually found under the upper eyelid after successful glaucoma surgery. It is formed by aqueous humour collecting under the conjunctiva.

carbonic anhydrase inhibitors. A class of drugs used either topically (e.g.,Trusopt) or orally (e.g., Diamox) to decrease intraocular pressure by inhibiting aqueous production. These drugs are related to the sulfonamides.

choroidal effusion. Choroidals are fluid-filled cyst-like areas formed at the back of the eye, usually within the first few weeks after glaucoma surgery, when the pressure is very low. They resolve as eye pressure increases. They are occasionally drained surgically to relieve a flat chamber.

chronic open-angle glaucoma. The most common form of glaucoma, occurring in over 90 per cent of all Caucasian patients with glaucoma. Also known as primary open-angle glaucoma.

ciliary block glaucoma. A very rare form of glaucoma that develops after glaucoma surgery. It is also called malignant glaucoma. It has nothing to do with cancer, and responds well to medical and/or surgical treatment.

ciliary body destructive procedure. The destruction of the ciliary body in order to decrease the production of aqueous humour and thereby lower pressure. This can be achieved by utilizing a freezing device (cryoprobe) or a laser (laser cyclocoagulation).

ciliary processes. Small finger-like organs found in the eye, responsible for the production of aqueous humour.

conjunctiva. The thin transparent membrane lining the sclera of the eye. It forms the lining of the bleb after a trabeculectomy.

cupping. An abnormal process that occurs within the optic nerve, often in association with high pressure. Cupping is associated with loss of nerve tissue in the optic nerve, leading to visual field loss.

deep sclerectomy. A surgical procedure used to lower intraocular pressure. In this procedure the eye is not entered, but rather is surgically manipulated on the surface.

diurnal tension curve. A test to determine the variation of intraocular pressure throughout the day. This variation is exaggerated in patients with glaucoma. Testing the pressure every one to two hours often allows for diagnosis of raised pressure.

flat chamber. A fairly common problem occurring after glaucoma surgery. It is due to excessive drainage of aqueous humour from the eye and is often associated with the formation of choroidal detachments. This condition is characterized by low eye pressure and contact between the iris and the cornea, and usually resolves with appropriate medical therapy. Surgical intervention is occasionally required.

fluorescein. A yellow-orange nontoxic dye that shines brightly in the presence of a special blue light. Fluorescein is placed in the eye before pressure is measured during tonometry.

frequency doubling perimetry. An easy, fast, and accurate visual field test used to screen new patients for glaucoma damage.

fundus photographs. Photographs taken of the optic nerve head as a baseline measure of the amount of cupping for future comparison.

glaucoma. Characteristic optic nerve and visual field loss often associated with raised pressure. The most common form is chronic or primary open-angle glaucoma.

glaucoma suspect. An individual with high intraocular pressure but without nerve cupping or visual field damage. A glaucoma suspect is also referred to as being ocular hypertensive.

hypotony. A situation where the eye is very soft. It develops after surgery and can be associated with a decrease in vision.

iritis. Inflammation of the coloured part of the eye (the iris). Also known as uveitis.

laser iridotomy. A procedure performed to prevent or cure angle-closure glaucoma.

laser trabeculoplasty. A laser procedure performed to lower intraocular pressure in patients with chronic open-angle glaucoma.

low-pressure glaucoma. An unusual form of glaucoma in which there is characteristic glaucoma nerve damage and visual field loss but a normal intraocular pressure. It is treated in the same way as chronic open-angle glaucoma.

malignant glaucoma. *See* ciliary block glaucoma.

miotics. A class of drugs that improve the flow of aqueous humour out of the eye. Miotics cause the pupil to become small, sometimes resulting in decreased vision. Headaches are a common side effect of these drugs.

Molteno/Ahmed/Baerveldt implant. One of the many different types of glaucoma drainage devices used after failed glaucoma surgery. It consists of a long tube inserted into the eye. The tube is attached to a base plate, which is stitched onto the sclera.

nasolacrimal occlusion. The application of pressure to the corner of the eye where two eyelids meet at the side of the nose. After application of drops, three minutes of nasolacrimal occlusion while keeping the eyelids closed will reduce systemic absorption of medication by up to 40 per cent. This will substantially reduce side effects, especially on the heart and lungs.

neovascular glaucoma. A rare form of glaucoma in which small blood vessels grow and cover the trabecular meshwork. Diabetes and retinal vein occlusion are the most common causes of this condition. This form of glaucoma is difficult to treat and is often associated with poor vision in the affected eye.

nerve fibre layer analyser (GDX). A newer imaging technique used to detect and evaluate retinal nerve fibre damage from glaucoma.

ocular hypertension. *See* glaucoma suspect.

optic nerve. The nerve that connects the back of the eye to the brain. Damage to this nerve is the cause of vision loss in glaucoma.

optical coherence tomograph (OCT). An imaging technique used to detect and evaluate the progression of retinal damage from glaucoma.

pigmentary glaucoma. An unusual form of glaucoma occurring in younger patients who are often mildly short-sighted. The iris releases pigment, which accumulates on various structures of the eye, including the trabecular meshwork. This form of glaucoma responds well to standard therapy and particularly to laser treatment.

primary open-angle glaucoma. *See* chronic open-angle glaucoma.

pseudoexfoliation. A form of glaucoma fairly common in older individuals, characterized by dandruff-like flakes of white material accumulating on various structures in the eye. The pressure is often high in patients with pseudoexfoliation, and this form of glaucoma often needs aggressive treatment. It responds well to the usual therapies, including laser treatment.

retinal vein occlusion. A blood clot in one of the small blood vessels at the back of the eye. Retinal vein occlusion can occur in patients with uncontrolled glaucoma. It can also cause a rare form of glaucoma called neovascular glaucoma.

scanning laser ophthalmoscopy (e.g., HRT). An imaging technique which uses a laser beam to capture three-dimensional images of the optic nerve head.

Schiötz tonometry. An older form of tonometry in which a metal device is placed on the eye while the patient is lying down.

sclera. The white, opaque outer lining of the eye, through which a trabeculectomy incision is made during glaucoma surgery.

sulfonamides. The class of drug to which the carbonic anhydrase inhibitors belong. Patients with sulfonamide allergies should not use these agents.

suture lysis. A laser procedure performed after trabeculectomy in which a scleral stitch is cut to allow for improved flow of aqueous humour from the eye. Successful suture lysis leads to improved bleb formation and lower intraocular pressure.

tonometer. A special device applied to the eye, commonly associated with a bright blue light, used to measure intraocular pressure. Glaucoma is usually diagnosed and monitored with Goldmann tonometry.

topical prostaglandins. A group of eye drops that improve the drainage of fluid from the eye through unconventional pathways.

trabecular meshwork. The drainage system of the eye that becomes blocked in glaucoma.

trabeculectomy. The most common surgical procedure used to lower intraocular pressure in patients with glaucoma.

transscleral cyclocoagulation. A laser procedure used to destroy the ciliary processes in patients with glaucoma.

uveitis. *See* iritis.

visual field. The range of peripheral vision, tested to both diagnose and monitor visual function in patients with glaucoma.

visual field test. A specialized vision test used to check the visual field of a patient with glaucoma. Humphrey, Octopus, and Dicon Perimeters are the pieces of equipment most widely used to test the visual field.